WILLIAM K. JOHNSTON III, MD

the PC diet

A MOTIVATIONAL GUIDE TO BETTER UNDERSTAND YOUR DIET, EXERCISE, AND THE PROTEIN TO CALORIE RATIO TO MAXIMIZE YOUR WEIGHT LOSS GOALS

FOR MORE INFORMATION ABOUT THIS BOOK:

BMED Press, LLC
5402 South Staples St.
Suite 200
Corpus Christi, Texas 78411
Phone: (817) 400 -1639
www.bmedpress.com

ISBN: 978-1-7349618-1-2

CONTENTS

Warning: Too much protein can be harmful and some people may lack the ability to digest protein, so consult with your doctor prior to this or any diet.

FOREWORD

INSPIRATION?

WHAT INSPIRES ME to write a book about a new diet? I guess it starts with my love for food—like a homemade wood-fired pizza! My problem, as it may be for others, was that I had reached the age and reduced activity levels that eating what I want, when I want, had resulted in weight gain. I've never had to worry much about weight in the past, but now I do! I realized, it was time to make a change, time to lose some weight, get in shape, and bring back some youth!

I first tried to increase my activity, a successful strategy used in my younger years, but I found myself fighting the numerous time constraints of family, work, and social commitments. When I did workout, I didn't get the weight losses I did 20 years ago. I finally had to accept, I'm older and cutting weight is tough and requires more than just adding some Activity of the Day (AOD). Sound familiar?

It was a time for a change. It was time for a diet! But what diet? So many diets, so many forbidden foods. And what about those special occasions (birthdays, tailgates, etc.) or dinner meetings, when I want to eat what everyone else is eating and drinking? At night, I look forward to sitting down with my wife and four boys and sharing the day's events over dinner. How can all this fit into a diet? Essentially, I wanted a diet to lose weight, but salvage some food freedom.

What I'll share in this book is my take on a diet, my approach to weight loss, and some strategies to losing weight. ***In no way does this book replace a visit and discussion with your personal physician on a diet that fits your health and goals.*** This book also focuses on weight loss, but doesn't address other aspects such as cholesterol, balanced nutrient intake, fiber, or a whole host of additional considerations. For starters, let's work on cutting calories and losing weight. At the very least, I hope this book inspires you to find the diet that works for you!

Misconceptions

Perhaps the other reason for writing a diet book was all the misconceptions about weight gain or loss I had found in the latest popular press, books, and in what I hear from my patients, acquaintances, friends or family members. Every few years, there's a new fad diet, one that is sure to help you lose weight and that will answer all your questions on weight loss, but they require you to eat foods in an awkward manner or completely eliminate foods you love (and there goes some serotonin release from your brain after one of your mom's warm, homemade, chocolate chip cookies).

Most diets are based on some particulars of leaving off foods you love and adding foods you don't. Some claim to boost metabolism, or avoid carbs, or worse yet, avoid fat (doesn't fat cause you to be fat?). **Essentially, many of these fad diets work, but they work for one primary reason, they help a person reduce the caloric intake more than the body requires, forcing the body into burning more calories than consumed.** In the beginning these fad diets work, but over time, most people can't withstand eating what just doesn't taste good or such a restrictive diet no one can stick to. What about a diet that is more flexible and one that the individual creates and adapts to personal needs and day-by-day social requirements? That's what I wanted.

As I researched diets, high protein diets and intermittent fasting made the most sense to me. After all, the body needs protein to rebuild and protein provides essentials to help the body in so many functions. However, protein does provide calories and too much protein can lead to too many calories, especially in some "high protein" shakes, foods, or supplements that also have high calories from carbohydrates (sugar), beyond that yielded from the protein. Intermittent fasting is a popular means to lose weight; by limiting food consumption to 8 hours a day, many people will limit calories and provide time for the body to burn reserves. Makes sense, but if one doesn't control calories, even within this smaller window, and calories consumed exceed calories burned, this diet will fail.

Vision

What I hope to share in this book is my simple solution to a diet and some basic strategies to increasing calorie burn. My goal was to make it short, concise, and a simple read for everyone. Throw the book in your travel bag, on your coffee table, or in your desk at work. Replace five minutes of looking at near-worthless information on your phone and read something that may empower you to change your life and turn back your biological clock! It is my hope that by reading this book, you'll learn how the body stores and loses weight, displace some common misconceptions, and *inspire you* to choose a diet or design a personal diet plan that works for you (check with your doctor before trying this or any diet). The PC Diet, therefore, is beyond a diet, it's about designing and personalizing your diet to fit your life, but not a diet eliminating all the food you love!

CHAPTER 1

INTRODUCTION

Simple, But Don't Overdo It!

IT SEEMS LIKE most diets are way too complex or really disruptive to your life. Do diets really need to be this difficult?

How simple can a weight control problem be? My Grandma's Approach.

My grandma had a weight control method she shared with me one day, unprovoked. As she ironed a pair of dated white pants in preparation for a summer event, she told me her secret. "You see these pants, I've had these since I got married. I try them on in the spring and if they are a little tight, then I know I need to eat a little less so they fit in the summer," she continued, "and I've been the same size since I was married and had kids… and I refuse to ever buy a bigger pair of pants." I never once saw my grandma on a special diet. I did see her eat chips with her lunch, have prime rib or a rack of lamb, or an occasional ice cream, but she never ate too much of any one thing, and I rarely saw her go back for seconds. She controlled her intake and reduced her intake if she needed to lose weight, but still ate a balanced diet of a variety of foods! Essentially, she portioned controlled and ate whatever she wanted, just not too much at any one time!

Furthermore, my Grandma chose a standard of weight that was acceptable to her and made her feel good, but she didn't overdo it; there is certainly something that should be said and cannot be stressed enough about too much weight loss being unhealthy!

Your body is programmed to have some fat energy reserves. The goal isn't to remove all those reserves, but to curb excess reserves and maintain a reasonable weight.

CHAPTER 2

SETTING GOALS AND THE BENEFITS OF WEIGHT LOSS

UNFORTUNATELY, THE REALITY is that if we look in the mirror, if we look at our friends, family, co-workers, or those in the community or even the stars in magazines, almost all of us could lose a few pounds. And this isn't just about image, more importantly, it's about our current and future physical and mental health. Our bones and joints have to carry the extra pounds and our heart and lungs work overtime to move weight. Additionally, for many, losing weight will light internal energy and drive… you can't help but feel better when you put on that pair of pants and see the waist too big or when you look in the mirror and see your youth return. Even more rewarding, is getting unsolicited comments from colleagues and friends on weight loss—now that's empowering! But you can't enjoy the downhill without putting some work and sacrifice into the uphill.

There are other benefits to weight loss. For example, in my medical practice, it is not uncommon for me to see men for low testosterone symptoms. In most of these patients, I encourage them to diet because excess fat can convert testosterone into estrogen. As men age, their testosterone production decreases. To compound this problem, when they carry more fat cells, testosterone conversion to estrogen increases. Less testosterone pulls men away from that adolescent/young man drive, and more estrogen further influences the loss of testosterone in a negative manner and causes more weight gain and less muscle formation. Women also have testosterone and small amounts of testosterone can positively influence a woman's body and mind, thus less testosterone from excess weight can negatively impact men and women.

Alternatively, put the car in reverse: lose fat and reduce testosterone conversion to estrogen. You may see more energy resulting in more activity. Now with more momentum, you have more weight loss and, perhaps, slow the aging process. You can avoid buying some "magic" natural pill that claims to boost your testosterone and build muscle, but really only lightens your wallet.

After all, as we age, what many of us want back from our youth is our energy, health, and image. Losing weight can help and may naturally increase relative testosterone levels.

I hear many people talking about wanting more muscle tone and mass. They start with weight training to get back some definition and add muscle. Unfortunately, building muscle takes time and a lot of work at the gym. Many of us don't have time to weight train and perform cardiovascular exercise, both of which are needed to optimize outcomes. Many of us already have muscle, the problem is the layer of fat camouflaging your muscle! One of the fastest ways to get more definition, is to take the blankets of fat off, revealing the muscle hiding below!

Losing weight doesn't necessarily mean getting down to some ideal body weight or to your youthful 20s weight. For most of us, even losing 10 pounds (lbs.) can make a tremendous difference physically and mentally. Should you set a realistic goal of losing 5% of body weight (that's 7.5 lbs. for a 150-lb person, and 10 lbs. for a 200-lb person, and 15 lbs. for a 300-lb person) and use this obtainable goal as a starting point to understanding diet? Absolutely!

Strategy: Lose 5% body weight, pause, and try to maintain this weight loss. Then reload and go for another 5%! Once you see the benefits, you'll buy in, but you need to stick with it for the first 5-10 lbs. When you see some changes, it recharges you to keep going. So, you've got this! Let's get to work, but first we need to understand some basics of how and why the body stores fat.

CHAPTER 3

WHY AND HOW YOUR BODY STORES AND LOSES FAT

Calories, Calories, Calories

WHAT IS THE key factor in losing weight? This can be a complex answer, or it can be a simple answer. Let's look at simple concepts, but it still comes down to calories!

Remove from your mind the thought that losing weight is simple or of the possibility that you can do something to make your brain turn on a switch to change your genetic make-up and suddenly burn more calories. Yes, people have different metabolisms (i.e., how fast their body digests food and burns calories) and some people are just programmed to store more or less fat regardless of the food they eat (good old genetics). It is completely unfair, but this genetic make-up (to this date) can't be altered. So, we need to detour around genetic headwinds and to tack to reach our goal.

You can't pick the genes that made you, so it's better to focus on the variables you can control.

Also, you can't trick your body into suddenly burning more calories. The possibility that certain foods cause your body to burn calories when digesting them or that "drinking water turns on something in your brain that makes you store less fat" is a stretch and, at best, could all be replaced by taking one flight of stairs or taking one less bite of food in a day!

It all really comes down to the fact that you must either increase your activity or eat fewer calories, or both! It's best to think of weight loss as 2-parts diet and 1-part exercise, so diet plays the greater role for most people.

It's best to think of weight loss as 2-parts diet and 1-part exercise, so diet plays the greater role in most people.

Losing weight isn't a complex formula. If you consume more calories than you burn, you will store this excess as fat and GAIN weight. If you consume less calories than you burn, you will LOSE weight. It's a mathematic equation:

Consumed Calories greater than Calories Burned = Weight gain

Burned Calories greater than Consumed Calories = Weight loss

Just as in real estate, location, location, and location are the 3 most important aspects to value, in dieting, it all comes down to 3 things.

It's all about CALORIES, CALORIES, and CALORIES.

So really, dieting can be as easy as balancing your caloric checkbook and controlling your calories!

Eat more calories than you burn, and you are storing fat. Burn more calories than you consume, and you will burn fat and lose weight. Your body doesn't know the difference between healthy or unhealthy foods, sugars, or fats, it only responds to how many calories the food brings. However, certain foods (sugars) can cause metabolic changes that may lead your body to crave more sugars and food. On the other hand, protein and some fats are beneficial in satisfying hunger for longer periods of time (vs. sugar). So, while the calories may be similar between a bite of sugar and bite of protein, the metabolic reaction of your body makes one less or more satisfied, respectively. But how do you control calories and how does timing of food intake play a role? For most of us, we need some help, and it starts with understanding the entire process of how the body stores and releases energy.

Understanding how the body stores and burns fat

A basic understanding of how the body stores and burns calories (or body fat in simple terms) is essential. It's all about survival, and you are programmed for saving for times of need. Our body stores energy in two primary forms and areas. One, as a form of glucose (i.e., sugars or carbohydrates) in the liver or muscle for immediate energy; and two, as fat, to be used when the liver or muscle stores are depleted.

Alternatively, if your liver is full of stored energy, then excess calories must be stored as fat cells. So, your body is always in a storing or burning mode, depending on its current state and need. If you always have high levels of glucose (i.e., sugars or carbohydrates) in your blood, the body doesn't burn liver reserves. If you don't burn liver reserves, you won't ever get to burning fat reserves. Essentially, you need a good 8- to 12-hour fast (not eating) and/or to burn enough stored glucose in the liver and muscle to deplete reserves and begin to spend body fat energy!

This concept of forcing the body into exhausting stored glucose and burning fat forms the basis of the popular fasting diet in which people are told to fast for 16 hours a day. This not only helps dip into fat reserves, but it also potentially eliminates a meal. When you can only eat for 8 hours a day, you can consume a good 750 calories per meal and get through the day with 1500 calories and stay on budget.

What makes you store fat?

Influences of time, health, post-pregnancy and genetics

During childhood and adolescence, or even in your younger (active!) adult years, your daily calorie needs are much greater. You are spending energy (calories) on growing or expending much more energy in your activities. Your metabolism slows down over time, and your body burns fewer calories as you get older and your lifestyle become more sedentary: sitting at your desk, on the couch, or while sleeping. As you age, all these things turn on you—you aren't growing, and you exchange that 1-hour basketball game or aerobic workout for picking kids up at school or sitting through long meetings. Your body just burns fewer and fewer calories (too much multimedia at your fingertips—get off the smart phone, unless you're reading this book!!!). Age is only one factor that may influence shifts in body weight.

Weight and Post-Pregnancy

Your body is programmed to store calories in case you need energy later, and pregnancy is the ultimate example of your body wanting to store calories so that you can provide constant energy to your baby. The demand for energy reserves results in a greater appetite in the second and third trimesters as more calories are needed for the substantial growth that takes place at this time. After giving birth, your body is still in a storing mode, but now you've adjusted eating habits to greater intake. These forces are now working against you, which makes losing the pounds more difficult.

Weight and Genetics

There are also genetics at work for or against you. People have different baseline metabolisms, different programs to store energy, and may absorb more or less of the calories they consume, which influences weight. Unfortunately, it's completely unfair, but your genetic makeup can't be changed, but the course can be altered and influenced by increasing activity: you must reduce calories consumed, otherwise, your body stores unused calories as fat.

You can't change your genetic makeup, but you can alter your intake and activity.

Therefore, the take home message:

Intake of calories exceeds calories burned = Stored Fat.

That's it!!!

So, to reduce body fat, you must figure out any eating pattern and activity pattern that keeps your calorie intake less than calories burned, and you will likely lose weight.

Stored Glucose = Liver + Muscle Reserves

Burn more calories than you take in and exhaust all glucose reserves, which forces the body to seek energy from fat reserves. Essentially, one needs to keep a caloric checkbook and know the balances.

A Deeper Understanding of How We Add Fat

One time I had a debate with a classmate in medical school. He wanted to lose weight, so he ate everything that said "nonfat" on it. He showed me a grocery bag of "nonfat" foods and told me he was going on a diet. He really believed that if it said "nonfat," it wouldn't make him fat. (I hope he learned more by the end of medical school!) However, he wasn't completely wrong: fatty foods (vs carbohydrates or protein) can cause fat storage because dietary fat equals greater calories per volume consumed.

Fat contains roughly 2x the calories as the same amount of protein or carbohydrates.

Fat is more calorie dense that proteins or carbohydrates. So, bite for bite, eating high-fat foods can make you fat easier because it results in twice the calories per bite. In other words, eating half as much of a high-fat food equals the same caloric intake as eating twice as much protein or carbohydrates. So fat intake doesn't necessarily make you fat, but too much fat can result in too many calories and this can get stored as… fat!!

The old saying "Once on the lips, twice on the hips" may be worth remembering. Fatty foods could be thought of as: one fat on the lips makes for 4x that on the hips!

CHAPTER 4

STEERING AROUND AND MINIMIZING INSTINCTIVE FOOD DESIRES AND SOCIAL FACTORS

THE TRUTH IS weight control centers on controlling calorie intake through learning portion control, timing your intake, and focusing on high protein diets that limit calories, yet keep you feeling "full" longer! But what other coping mechanism can you use for times you need to slip off your diet or you are going to have foods high in carbs? You just need to find a way to control the calories you put into your body, which means asking yourself' "Is this (food or drink) worth the calories? Is there an alternative with fewer calories? For example, specialty beer equals 300+ calories vs light beer, which equals 100 calories; is that specialty beer worth the extra calories? You get to decide if it is worth dipping into your daily caloric budget!

Ask yourself if the food or drink is worth the calories?

Some people have no trouble changing bad habits, but slipping into instinctive behavior and our natural responses to familiar foods (comfort foods) is a battle. Furthermore, controlling calories isn't easy because of physiologic, psychological, and social influences. Your body is programmed to store energy for times of need. This instinct has been passed down for generations and is deeply embedded to ensure survival during times of scarcity.

For many people, eating high calorie foods feels good, releasing endorphins, and often curbing emotional downturns. For most of us, eating often is a social activity with friends, workers, or family. For business, a meeting over a coffee or dinner at a restaurant can be necessary, but these are usually high-calorie events! So, how can we control this intake and minimize the draw on our daily caloric checkbook? Better yet, can we learn techniques to burn calories when we need to lose weight and also learn to control caloric intake while using exercise to supplement weight control? Can we make room for our afternoon snack, gourmet anniversary dinner, or tailgate party? What we really need is an adjustable and personalized diet. We have a budget of our daily caloric intake, and we need to work within that budget to attain and maintain a healthy weight.

Essentially, dieting involves planning for the future and keeping a balanced caloric intake. Can we balance eating weaknesses with strengths and learn to save calories for a planned overconsumption?

We save for vacation. Why not save up for a special meal?

Analogous to saving up for a vacation, if you want to go for a special dinner or work dinner, you need to save up some calories (e.g., cut your afternoon calories) or do an extra activity (e.g., burn some extra calories) before the meeting (or both!). It's always easier to have the cash to pay for the vacation ahead of time than to try to pay off the credit card debt after the trip.

Working in anticipation of a reward is always easier than working to pay off a previous expenditure. Why treat caloric intake differently? Prepare for the caloric intake before and then enjoy the reward!

However, we all know spending sprees happen and must be paid off. So, if you do binge one night, make sure you get to work immediately to pay off those calories with an evening activity (walk, hit the hotel gym, and/or whatever activity can burn some calories before bed-oh yeah!). Alternatively, or additionally, the day after, increase your activity and reduce your intake—all to maintain a balanced caloric checkbook!

Life is full of challenges and temptation, these can act as headwinds to obtaining your weight loss goals. Don't let these winds knock you off course!

- **Want to learn more about how the body stores and burns fat, go to the next page, Chapter 5.**
- **Ready to get started with the PC Diet, go to Chapter 6.**

CHAPTER 5

HOW DOES OUR BODY HANDLE FATS, PROTEINS, AND CARBOHYDRATES?

THE HUMAN BODY is programmed to store unused energy. The body breaks almost everything you eat into components that can be used or stored. So, let's look at *carbohydrates, fats, and protein.* This can be complex, but in simple terms, it's worth understanding! For a little more technical details, read the italic print.

Carbohydrates

In simple terms, carbohydrates come from foods high in sugar (sweets, breads, and pasta.). The body stores carbohydrates in the liver and muscles. When needed, the body activates theses reserves. The pancreas is the organ that acts as the "crossing guard" that controls if the body is in a storing mode or a burning mode. When more energy is needed, the pancreas tells the body to burn the stored energy. Alternatively, the pancreas can tell the body to store more energy to replenish reserves. The pancreas responds to carbohydrates (sugar) and shifts the body into a storing mode. However, if the liver and muscles are already full of stored energy, the body diverts the extra energy to back-up storage in the form of FAT! So too much carbohydrates (sugar) that isn't needed gets turned into fat. Worse yet, carbohydrates activate the pancreas to sends signals that tells the brain that the body needs energy and this leads to the signal for eating- which then leads craving more sugar! This is why carbohydrates are minimized in diets and too much carbohydrates play a major role in obesity.

A more technical description in italic below:

(Carbohydrates are converted into glucose, which is a form of energy used by cells. When glucose is released into your circulation, the pancreas stops releasing glucagon, which normally causes the body to breakdown fats into energy, and releases insulin, which causes your body to store glucose as a reserve called glycogen. Glycogen is primarily stored in the liver. When glucose levels are low, insulin levels are low, and the body responds by releasing stored glucose from the liver. Glucose can also be stored in muscles, which use glucose for energy).

The liver and muscle cells have a maximum storage ability of glucose (as glycogen), so excess glucose (sugar, carbs) that can't be stored is sent to the liver for conversion into fat (fatty acids-triglycerides).

So excess glucose that isn't used or stored as glycogen turns into body FAT. This is one source of body fat. Consuming too much dietary fat, results in excess calories, which also gets stored as fat.

Fats:

Fatty acids (fats) are broken down by the body into useful components that help build cells and function within cells of the body, but they also produce more than 2x the energy or adenosine triphosphate (ATP; the technical name for the energy "currency" that is used in the body) as do protein or carbohydrates.

So, in basic terms, for every spoon of fat you eat, you could eat 2 spoons of protein or carbohydrates and equal the same amount of energy (calories). Excess fat produces triglycerides, which end up adding to fat storage. Triglycerides and cholesterol can have harmful effects on the body (blood vessels) that are beyond the scope of this book, but in terms of calories, they may harm the calorie count by the simple fact of double the energy compared with carbohydrates or protein.

Protein

Protein is found in meat, dairy products, nuts, tofu, combined grains and legumes, etc. and is broken down into amino acids. There are twenty amino acids that are essential for various functions, including building muscle and regulating the immune system. The human body can only synthesize eleven of these amino acids, the other nine are considered *essential amino acids.* These essential amino acids cannot by synthesized by the human body, and must be obtained through dietary protein. Once broken down into amino acids, they are used to repair cells or for the production of new cells.

One important thing to know is that excess amino acids and proteins cannot be stored in the body and must be safely excreted. In the liver, excess amino acids are converted to ammonia, which is toxic if not reduced to urea and water, which is released into the bloodstream and then filtered by the kidneys to safely pass out of the body as urine. – In other words, you pee it out.

When your body needs energy, it initially reaches for stored energy (glucose) in the liver and muscle. After glucose is depleted, the body looks to fat reserves, and finally, to breaking down muscle protein, as a source of energy in long-term starvation circumstances.

Consumed protein, unlike carbohydrates, does not activate the body into a storage mode. Alternatively, when you eat sweets, sugars (carbs), your body sends a signal to release insulin to store the sugar. But higher insulin levels drop your blood sugar levels and the brain senses this and sends a signal for you to eat more sugars. It's a negative cycle that feeds on itself. Protein, however, does not cause release of insulin and, through complex transmitters to the brain, provides messages to your brain that you have eaten enough. This is why many people notice that eating a breakfast full of sugars causes them to feel hungry shortly after vs one that is mainly of proteins that fulfills them through the morning!

<u>A word of caution, there may be risk with consuming too much protein.</u> Although no major studies link high protein to kidney damage in people with normal-functioning kidneys, people with preexisting kidney disease may be susceptible to kidney harm. High protein diets can cause calcium loss through the kidney, which can deplete the body of calcium, but also

increase the calcium in the urinary tract, increasing the risk of creating kidney stones.

Protein requirements vary depending on physical activity and growth (and one's other health conditions). In general, adults can look at a minimal daily average of 0.3-0.5 grams per pound of lean body weight (although up to 1 gram per pound is often used for athletes, heavy exercisers). For most people, a good goal is 100 grams of protein per day.

WARNING: *A rare disorder of an inability to digest proteins does exist (Lysinuric Protein Intolerance) and is most commonly seen in people of Finnish and Japanese origin. People with this disorder must restrict protein intake and/or take medications to help eliminate excess nitrogen. Failure to remove the waste products of protein digestion can lead to seizures, coma, and death.*

CHAPTER 6

PROTEIN-TO-CALORIE SCORE: "PC SCORE"

PROTEIN IS RESPONSIBLE for repairing your body and rebuilding muscle broken down during exercise. Protein also takes more time to breakdown and many people feel that high protein diets lead to less hunger problems. Today, many stores sell "protein bars" or health clubs sell "protein shakes." Are these good? Yes and No.

What you want to do is maximize your protein intake with minimizing the calories. So, head out to the store and look at all the protein bars. There are some that give you 21 grams of protein, but 400 calories and others that give you the same grams of protein, for half the calories. Protein shakes? Some provide 20 grams of protein for 200 calories and some cost you 400-800 calories!

What's the take home? I like to think of how much protein am I getting for the calories consumed. So, protein, divided by calories, multiplied by 100 equals the PC Score. It's all about the PC Score. (Time to pull out the phone and use the calculator or learn to estimate in your head).

Protein/calories x 100 = PC Score

Protein (in grams) divided by calories, multiplied by 100

So, take out your phone,

Enter the grams of protein on any label or menu.

Divide by the number of calories on any label or menu.

Multiple by 100.

This is the PC Score.

If a protein shake has 20 grams of protein and 200 calories, enter in 20, divide by 200 and multiple by 100= 10. This shake has a PC Score of 10 (Great!).

If a protein shake has 20 grams of protein and 400 calories, enter 20, divide by 400 and multiple by 100= 5. This shake has a PC Score of 5 (Good).

What might not be as obvious, are some foods you might eat at a restaurant or picking up a snack. What can you choose on the menu to maximize the PC Score?

Roast beef sandwich: 23gm protein, 360 calories or Chicken Sandwich: 14g and 400 calories? Let's calculate the PC Score:

Roast beef: 23/360 x 100 = 6.3 (Good!)

Chicken Sandwich: 14/400 x 100 = 3.5 (Poor!)

What about a burger with no dressing and ½ the bun?

21 grams of protein and 300 calories: PC Score

PC score: 21/300 x 100 = 7

Other common foods with high PC Scores:

Can of tuna fish: 20gm protein, 90 calories: 20/90 x 100 = 22 (PC Score 22!)

Milk: 8gm protein, 120 calories: 8/120 x 100 = 6.7.

Common foods with low PC Scores:

French Fries: 3gm protein, 350 calories: 3/350 x 100 = 0.8 (Bad!)

Bagel/cream cheese: 14gm protein, 436 calories: 14/436 = 3.2 (There are better choices!)

PC Scores of more than 5 are great. Start to get a list of foods and snacks with high PC Scores! These are more likely to satisfy hunger for longer periods of time.

Next, start keeping a list of foods with high PC Scores. For example, an egg white has one of the highest PC Scores. It has 4 grams of protein for 17 calories and the PC Score of 24! (caution: consuming too many egg whites can cause a loss of biotin and be harmful to your health). Hotels frequently have breakfast bars with a bowel full of boiled eggs. Grab a few eggs, harvest the egg whites, season with pepper, and this is a tasty snack or breakfast! I like to make "Dirty Egg Whites"- which means I removed most all of the yolk and leave just a small amount of yolk on the egg for taste. What if you eat the entire egg? An egg has 6 grams of protein for around 70 calories. This results in a PC Score of 8.6, but egg yolks do have cholesterol, which can be harmful.

A glass of 2% milk has a PC Score of 6.7- so yes, a glass of 2% milk is actually a benefit to your diet. Some protein shakes are good and some have too many calories. One protein milk product has 25 grams of protein per 160 calories; this amounts to a PC Score of 16! What about Tofu? It has 8 grams of protein for 70 calories and the PC Score of 11; it also provides all the essential amino acids! So, although limiting calories can help a person lose weight, we also must consider the body's need for protein, but consuming it doesn't have to be a lot of extra calories, as long as you choose wisely and choose foods with high PC Scores.

PC Score Goal: Above 5!

<5:	Bad
5-10:	Good
10-15:	Great
>15:	Super

CHAPTER 7

LET'S GET STARTED WITH THE PC DIET!

The basics of getting started with the PC Diet

GETTING STARTED: FIRST *and foremost, the caution: Consult with and follow the advice of your physician before starting any diet. This is only a summary of how I designed a diet for me. This eating plan may be harmful to some with specific health issues, known or not known. You may also consider consulting with your physician to design a plan that is safe for you.* But here are some general concepts and considerations:

1. Commit to losing weight: Write yourself a card with your 30-day goal. Place this card on your refrigerator and on your phone's screen saver! Alternatively, challenge a friend or family member to join you with a weight loss goal.
2. Set a goal for the first month and a final goal (5% of current weight for first month)
3. Buy a scale
4. Get a friend to support you
5. Join a diet club on social media
6. Read this book and understand the basics
7. Get started!
8. Make the challenge fun!

Getting started: Desire, drive, and setting obtainable goals!

Certainly, one of the first requirements is to want to lose weight. It sounds obvious, but isn't always. We need self-motivation and, if you can't find this, then you need a buddy system to help you (another option is to spend a bunch of money on a diet coach). You need to take a look in the mirror and reflect back on some old photos. Some of us may not realize that we have some pounds to lose, so we don't even try. Many of us still imagine ourselves in our youthful bodies and are in a state of denial, thinking we still look good and failing to see the extra pounds on our belly or showing in our face or on our legs. For some of us, life changes and challenges led to weight gain, and family or work requirements make us think we don't have time to worry about our weight. Some of us don't see the slow change, we make excuses to justify the changes, or we get hung up on the fact that we've never had to worry about what we ate or our weight. Some of us realize we need to lose some weight, but we just can't do it. Last, some make honest efforts by engaging in daily exercise programs, but without a reduction in calories, they fail to lose weight (and many times people even increase their intake when they start exercise programs),

The truth is, most people start weight loss programs by increasing their activity, but wipe out any gains by increasing their caloric intake. You get more results from reducing caloric intake than by exercising. Perhaps the best combination is that any weight loss program depends on 2/3 diet modification and 1/3 increased activity!

Now let's get started!

Buy a scale. This is the first and most important step. Nothing fancy, but something for a daily weight check. It's best to check your weight at the same time each day. In the morning, after getting out of bed provides the best time for consistent measurements. Use the bathroom, remove all your clothes, and step on the scale before your shower. Weights can vary with simple things like hydration (or lack of it) and constipation, but over time, these variables average out. Occasionally, you can weigh yourself after work or in the evening at bedtime; compare evening vs morning weight to see how different times of day can yield slightly different values. You often have a net water loss at night (because you don't eat or drink at night, but your kidneys filter the blood and remove water). Furthermore, at night, with caloric control, you are burning some calories as you sleep, and hopefully dipping into fat reserves!

The body needs water and drinking water throughout the day is beneficial to many aspects of health. But it should be remembered for day to day variations, that the old saying of "a pint a pound" should be remembered. If you drink a 16-ounce glass of water or don't empty your bladder of 16oz, this appears as another pound on the scale in the morning. It's all relative, but keep it simple: empty your bladder and weigh yourself before eating or drinking in the morning. This will minimize factors that may swing your weight day by day. (BTW: for many, drinking a glass of water before bed and after the morning weigh-in is a great way to start your day!)

Simple measure, simple goal:

There are other ways to measure weight loss beside a scale. Get an old pair of pants that you can get on, but just barely button. Use these as one of your goals. Each month, put on the pants and see how they fit! Or find a belt, tighten and mark it, recheck monthly. There's nothing more rewarding than needing to buy a new pair of pants because the old ones are falling off!

Estimated Daily Calories

Because we now know it all comes down to maximizing protein and minimizing calories (PC Score), and that if we consume too many calories, we gain fat, and if we burn more than we take in, our bodies will burn fat, then we need to know about daily limits. Fortunately, there are numerous apps and websites to help you calculate your daily caloric needs. These are based on sex, weight, height, age, and even adjusted for daily activity levels. In the perfect world, you calculate this daily caloric need and attempt to reduce your calculated daily caloric intake by 500 calories. In doing so, you should lose about a pound per week (it's estimated that a reduction of 3000 calories will equal one pound of weight loss; so, reducing daily caloric intake by 500 calories/day for 6 to7 days should result in a reduction of 3000 calories/

week and a 1-lb loss in a week). Most moderately active adult women age 19-50 years need about 2000 calories per day; moderately active women older than age 50 need about 1800 calories per day. Moderately active men age 18-45 years need about 2600 calories per day; moderately active men age 45 to 65 need about 2400 calories per day; and moderately active men older than age 65 need about 2200 calories per day.

In the perfect world, one calculates the daily caloric need and attempts to reduce daily calories by 500. Once you save a total of 3000 calories in a week, you should lose at least a pound a week!

But I like a far simpler approach. Think about what you usually consume every day. Let's find a way to cut your calories with a general goal of consuming around 1500 calories in a day for the average adult (most adults consume around 2500 calories/day and cutting to 1500, yields 2 lbs. per week!). That would give you 400 calories to spend on breakfast, 700 on lunch, 150 on an afternoon snack and then 250 for dinner if you are cutting mainly at night (an effective means). Alternatively, if you value dinner with your family or business contacts, you may reduce your calories during the day and spend 250 on breakfast, 500 on lunch, and then leave 750 calories for dinner. Have a big dinner event, save calories through the day, skip breakfast, lunch (500), exercise (-250) and you have 1250 to spend at dinner. All in all, these all add up to 1500!

Not all dinners out have to be high-calorie meals and drinks can add significant calories to any night out. If you wanted an alcoholic beverage, an ultralight beer cuts the calories by almost a 1/3 compared with many microbrews (I recently discovered a great Italian beer with only 120 calories). It all comes down to checking labels and making choices. Additionally, avoid the greasy appetizers, skip the bread, and minimizing the sides (like mashed potatoes); limit yourself to the main dish. After all, even a petit filet at a major steakhouse only costs you ~340 calories and provides almost 40 grams of protein (PC Score of 40/340 x 100 = 12). Most menus show calories and many times our minds are warped on what has more calories. The chef's salad with meats and cheese provides relatively low protein and cost you more calories than a steak. A quick search on your phone can estimate protein and calories for you if they are not on the menu.

So, your job is to figure out how to maximize your protein and budget out your calorie goal for the day. A candy bar is all sugar and sets you back 200 to 300 calories (and high sugars can lead to high insulin release and may cause you to feel hungry soon after). A protein bar tastes like a candy bar, can provide 12 grams of protein at only a cost of 200 calories with a PC Score=6 and may be a better snack!).

In the same breath, not all "protein snacks" are good. For example, a protein smoothie sounds like a good snack, but many of these contain a lot of carbs - most damaging, they push 400-600 calories. Want a healthier snack with protein, stop and get some 2% milk (which contains 6 grams of protein for only 120 calories, PC Score of 5!). An apple sounds healthy as well as a snack and it does contain some vitamins and fiber, but an apple has 95 calories and no protein. It's a good snack, but you can see why it's so important to focus the PC Score. The protein is used by your body for repairs and building muscle, so protein is important, but the calories are what influence fat burning or storage.

Really, just cutting 500-750 calories/day will likely shed 2 lbs./week in most people! Eat high protein foods to satisfy your hunger and help save calories!

So, the PC Diet essentially comes down to maximizing the protein for the cost of the calories in the food you eat. That's it, and it can work!

CHAPTER 8

WORKING OUT TO LOSE WEIGHT?

Can't I just workout and lose weight? ("I'm working out, but not losing weight;" "I got busy and couldn't workout, so I gained it back;" "I've actually gained weight since starting my workouts, but my trainer says it's from muscle I'm adding"- Do these sound familiar???

Working out is a great way to supplement any diet and weight loss program. But we have many hours during the day to burn additional calories with our day-to-day activities. In fact, changing activity doesn't necessarily mean spending an hour at the gym or running 6 miles. Many of us don't have the time to do this and many "working out" activities don't really burn that many calories or burn less than what you can accomplish in your day-to-day activities (although exercise has other benefits than burning calories, such as cardiovascular health, release of endorphins, and social interactions). Worse yet, the best activities at the gym that burn the most calories are usually the least desirable. Running and rowing, for example, burn significant calories, but even these activities, must be maintained for 60 min to burn off an average meal. For most all of us, burning off some fat is the fastest and most effective means to improve one's body definition. You have muscle there, you just need to wipe off some coverings!

Walking backwards out of the gym?

Most gym workouts don't burn as many calories as you may think, especially if they don't include cardiovascular exercise (although cross-fit does address both a cardio aspect and a muscle workout). Remember, cutting calories is key. Go walk on the treadmill briskly for an hour and see how much that burns (250-300 calories); run a 3K at 7 min pace and you might burn 400 calories. Now stop at the gym's nutrition center and order a protein shake… it taste good, you feel good, having just sweated and worked out for an hour, but now you have added 400 to 600 calories. Protein is good for rebuilding muscles, but what else is going on in that shake? Now look at the calories burned during your workout, 250, 300? Better yet, stop at a chain juice company, consume a protein shake and get a "healthy" looking pretzel (now you are at over 800 calories) and heading the wrong direction for losing weight. You actually would have lost more weight staying on your couch at home.

Skip the protein shake and stop for a celebratory specialty coffee after your workout? You just added 400+ calories back. These are all big-ticket items that seem healthy or innocent, but really cut into your calorie budget for the day or worst yet, zero out all your hard work for the day! There's nothing wrong with a low calorie (300 cal.) protein shake or coffee, but this has to replace a meal! You get to choose, but you need to balance and limit your caloric intake. You can choose the specialty coffee, but that must count as a meal and satisfy you or you need to do an activity to gain room for those calories. It also contains little protein, has a low PC Score, and will likely provide only short-term satisfaction.

As you start to think in these terms, making choices about foods, you start to ask questions like, "is that worth the calories"? Also, if I need a snack, let's pick a high PC Score snack (PC Score >5).

Burning calories is determined by how much work you do. This is dependent on how much weight you're moving, how far you move it, and how fast you do it. The more you move during your walk, the more you burn; so, using walking sticks or arm exercises burns more calories. You are awake for almost 16 hours a day. Use this time to increase your distance and speed of how fast you walk make a difference (so walk briskly around the office, park at the back of the lot, and take the stairs!)

The calories burned by day-to-day activities add as many, if not more, than a 1-hour intense gym workout!!!

Take a simple look at identical twins A and B that weigh the same: Twin A walks 1 hour at the gym at 3.5 mph and burns around 300 calories, but sits at a desk for 8 hours and lives a sedentary life once home. Twin B doesn't go to the gym, but walks 10 minutes a day taking the kids to the bus stop, walks for 15 minutes at the start of lunch hour, and takes the stairs throughout the day to business meetings. Twin B burns the same 300 calories and never stops at the gym. Certainly, working out has other health benefits, e.g., cardiovascular benefits, helps release endorphins that makes you feel good, and supplements normal day activity. But the stop at the gym is generally thought of as the only means to lose weight when many times the net benefit is little if not used with an effective decrease in caloric intake, or, at the very least, not counter-balanced by increased caloric intake after a workout (Don't Walk Out of the Gym Backwards!).

Emptying the reserves

Any type of muscle use can burn the stored energy (glucose) in the muscles and this serves as the basis for increasing your activity, no matter how small or large. In reality, small activities are done in much higher volume than the trip to the gym and ends up burning a bulk of the calories. Those choices you make during the day to take the stairs, walk briskly (versus casually), and move more can all add up.

Your weight affects the calories you burn during any activity; e.g., a person of average weight (e.g., a 5'5" women weighting 130 lbs. or a 5'10" man weighing 176 lbs.) will burn fewer calories than someone who is overweight—carrying that extra weight uses more energy (calories). But let's look at an example: if you climb the stairs at work and complete 10 flights of stairs in a day, this equates to approximately 100 calories. Another calorie-burning tip is to park your car at the back of the lot at work and add a brisk 10-minute walk to and from work, and you may burn another 100 calories. Just with these two simple life changes, you could burn 200 calories. Double these tasks and you have burned 400 calories! You can use these extra calories for weight loss or use these to cancel out an excess intake of calories…it's all about keeping that caloric checkbook balanced.

The bottom line, working out at the gym can be very beneficial, but there are many ways to increase your caloric burn if you don't have time to stop at the gym! Just take the longest walk and the stairs to the next meeting!

Exercise burns energy stores in muscle and provides a sink hole for calories consumed after working out. Avoid the rebound eating after a good gym workout, which is a common cause of lack of weight loss, even if you are working out daily.

CHAPTER 9

ACTIVITY OF THE DAY (AOD) AND "I CAN'T RUN"

ONCE CLEARED BY your doctor, adding an activity of the day (AOD) is important. This adds calories that you can consume or add to weight loss. The best way to start is to commit to 20 minutes per day of some activity for one month. An AOD can be a sport, but the easiest activity to incorporate into your daily life is walking. Maintaining this commitment can be challenging, but with a plan, you can do it: Start with doing your chosen activity for at least 20 minutes per day for one month. For most of us, this is very easy to work into our daily lives, but can become a greater challenge when things outside of day-to-day life are factored in; for example, when travelling—this can present an even greater challenge. But you can do it: arrive at the hotel with only half an hour before a meeting? Get in a short walk, turn on some music, get out, and get it over with it! If your AOD is a sport, consider walking/running as a viable substitute when traveling—it's easier to work into your schedule at a hotel, but go back to your sport when you return home. Many people get a lunch hour; what a perfect time to get in some exercise for 30 minutes.

And walking can turn into running, if you want it to. True, running isn't for everyone, and some people have health conditions that limit their ability to take on running. Most people, however, don't run because it's plain out simply no fun… in the beginning. But once you learn to do it, the powerful endorphins post-workout really do make you feel good, have more energy, and help you sleep well. Running burns twice the calories as walking and because you cover twice the distance, for equal 20 min workout, you get nearly 4 times the workout and caloric burn. But most people just can't get themselves to start. So how do you do it?

First, and I can't say this often enough, you must make sure your doctor clears you to do any workout, exercise, or run. Next, you start with an obtainable goal, and you make it a daily routine for at least 1 to 2 months.

To begin, start walking, and then progress. When you want to walk faster, just pick a portion of your walk to pick up the pace for a set distance (e.g., pick one block, or the end of the road, or "make it to the Smith's mailbox"), then pick up the pace until the goal is reached (this is called an interval or Fartlek training—an old Swedish term that means "speed play"). As you improve, you can do more intervals during your walk and soon advance to adding short jogs for short distances or goals. Soon you can do more jogging intervals and eventually work up to doing more jogging than walking and eventually running, then running longer distances.

What about those days I want to skip my walk or run? There will always be those days when you get home tired or just can't get out of bed. The best way to attack these days is to talk yourself into doing a shortened version of your normal workout. If you normally walk 3 miles, tell yourself that you are going to just go walk 1/2 mile. Most of the time, when you get out there, you'll start to feel better and push through to a lot more than a 1/2 mile and many times reach your daily distance goal. Learning to convince your mind and body into working out when you don't feel like it is a key development in weight control and exercise. Most of the time, your body has the energy to move, it's your mind that's stagnant. Lastly, the first few minutes of a run always feels tough until the body gets warmed up…so fight through this time and don't quit! Exercise will empower you and recharge you!

A workout can help you rebound from overeating or help you avoid overindulging, once you train yourself to think in terms of caloric intake versus output: "If I eat that bowl of ice cream, I'll need to exercise 20 more minutes to work it off." Okay, none of us are perfect, and you enjoy yourself one night at dinner. You get home and start dreading the morning's scale report. This is the time to put your shoes on, get on the treadmill or out the door and do some extra exercise before bed. (Please note, any activity before going to sleep burns calories—dieting can be fun-time to diet with your mate?) Alternatively, get up early and get in an extra walk or run! Last, if you know a big calorie dinner is coming (work meeting or celebration dinner), budget in a 30-minute workout or run to free up some calories for dinner! Basically, we are budgeting our calorie intake and if we need a bigger budget, we need to put some work in to have room!

CHAPTER 10

DIET PHASES: CHOOSE, MODIFY, USE THE DIET PLAN THAT WORKS FOR YOUR GOALS

Burning/Maintenance/Gaining

Burn Phase: *aggressive implementation of low-calorie intake with the goal of dropping weight.*

Dinner-Time Burn Phase

The DINNER-TIME BURN PHASE is used to lose fat or to maintain a weight. So, there are two aspects. The first involves a set time (a month, a season) to actively pursue losing weight. It is best to pick a month of the year and follow the diet strictly. Think about planning to have a light dinner (250 cal.) most nights. Maybe this means 4 nights vs 3, maybe this means 6 nights of 7. It all depends on your goals. It's probably best to keep it reasonable and shoot for 4 to 6 nights of a light dinner and give yourself the reward of a dinner out (just don't overdo it!). Have a midweek work or birthday dinner? Then alter your daily intake to make room for a dinner, and don't overeat. During the Burn Phase, during that month, give the diet your full attention. Try to get 12 hours of fasting (so, perhaps you eat a late dinner at 7 p.m. and don't eat again until 7 a. m.). After this month, you can choose to continue in the Burn Phase or switch to the Maintenance Phase.

Simple Dinner-Time Burn Plan							
Meal	Mon	Tues	Wed	Thurs	Fri	Sat	Sun
Break-fast	normal	normal	normal	normal	normal	late BF	late BF
Lunch	normal	normal	normal	normal	normal	None	None
Dinner	250 cal.	250 cal.	250 cal.	250 cal.	Dinner	Early Dinner	Early Dinner

(BF = Breakfast)

Day Time Burn Phase

Alternatively, pick the DAYTIME BURN PHASE, where you save calories during the day. Eat some egg whites and a glass of milk for breakfast (200 cal.), eat a 20 gram protein bar with a large water for lunch (200 cal.), after-noon snack (apple (100 cal.) or protein bar (200 cal.), eat an early dinner with your family or business associates (600-800 cal.)—Now you end your day with around 1100 to 1300 calories (you can modify all these and take in regular food, but limit calories during the day to allow for a regular dinner at night). However, you can do it, staying under 1500 calories, which for most adults is a typical goal.

Simple Day Time Burn Plan							
Meal	Mon	Tues	Wed	Thurs	Fri	Sat	Sun
Break-fast	< 300	< 300	< 300	< 300	< 300	None	None
Lunch	< 400	< 400	< 400	< 400	< 400	< 600	< 600
Snack	100	100	100	100	100	100	100
Dinner	< 700	< 700	< 700	< 700	< 700	< 700	< 700
Total calories	< 1500	< 1500	< 1500	< 1500	< 1500	< 1500	< 1500

Maintenance Phase:

During the maintenance phase, you calculate your caloric intake to avoid weight gain (you can use one of many apps). You can still carry the goal of 1500 calories, with some days allowing up to 2000 or more, depending on activity and scale changes. During this month, you are just trying not to give back the weight you lost the month before. Perhaps you get motivated within the maintenance month to mix in a week or two of low-calorie dinners or Day Time Burns. Perhaps you look to a substitute light dinner that provides fewer calories (250). For example, tofu or a piece of grilled chicken breast and a water (<250 calories) or an apple (95 calories) and yogurt (100 calories)). Protein bars can be found with 12 to 16 grams of protein and around 200 calories. This makes for a great meal with a big glass of water! (But remember… Some protein bars harbor 400+ calories and may not be a great choice). Calculate the PC Score!

Maintenance Phase: ***normal diet resumes while avoiding high–caloric intake or alternating low-calorie intake, with no weight gain or loss is observed.***

Most people's weight will vary by day, but it's the day-by-day trend that determines long-term outcomes. If you see the scale creeping up, adjust your calories down and/or activity up – better to do both!

How Can A Fast Fit In?

There is some importance to the 12 to 16 hours fast (fast = not eating food, only water). Your body needs to be challenged to deplete all the energy reserves stored within the liver. The body will then go to the stored energy of fat cells. It is usually easiest to fast at night, when you are sleeping, when your mind doesn't sense hunger. Changing your mind set to go to bed a little hungry isn't easy, but when you realize that you can wake up and be lighter by just getting to bed, this becomes more rewarding. Waking up hungry, with your stomach growling, at first seems unnerving, but soon you realize that your body is sending signals that the liver ran low, and the body was likely turning to fat.

The Fast Followed by a Morning Burn:

Want to enhance the fat burn or make room for a nice brunch with family or friends? Wake up (hopefully a little hungry), drink a glass of water, and get yourself out on a brisk walk for 15 to 30 min (or better yet a run!!). The body is forced to keep breaking down fat. (*Again, get your doctor approval and this may not be acceptable for all people's health conditions!*) A morning workout before eating is a great way to start out a weekend and the endorphins generated from a morning run, coupled with stepping on the scale and seeing a difference will fuel your enthusiasm for more! Again, it's about teaching your body and mind to learn what it needs to do to lose or maintain weight, but still eating the foods you love!!!

Other Diet Strategies To Cut Calories: Money Method:

Find some "play money" at the local dollar store or siphon off some game money tucked away in a closet. If your daily goal is 1500 calories, find fifteen 100's (or 15 silver dollars or make some diet bills) and put them in your wallet or purse. This is what you have to spend for the day. You can round to the nearest 100 to keep it simple. So, you eat a protein bar and black coffee for breakfast ($300 dollars), you eat a light lunch ($300), you have a vegetable/fruit snack or protein bar or milk ($100) in the afternoon, and now you have $800 (i.e., 800 calories) left in your wallet for dinner with your family! Alternatively, you have a specialty coffee and pastry (600), sandwich/chips and lemonade (600), protein snack size bar (100), now you have only 300 left for dinner (i.e., you need to eat a light dinner!). Obviously, after a few days of this, you can keep track of your spending in your head for the day, but a simple system like this can help you track approximate calories for the day. Not sure how many calories are in a food? Pull out your phone and search it, it's probably there! Your days can vary and you can find which eating method helps keep you under your calorie goal, but generally maximizing protein and minimizing calorie per bite (PC Score) will provide the best method for staying on budget.

Personalize your diet.

A weight loss diet that works is a diet that reduces caloric intake and results in weight loss. A successful weight loss diet is sustainable, rather than a fad diet of awkward foods that sooner or later you abandon. Therefore, you need to find a diet that works for you—whatever way you can control your calories! Additionally, you need to make daily or weekly adjustments when the weight breaks a set threshold.

The PC Diet, therefore, is a concept that teaches you how to balance the caloric checkbook, emphasize the value of protein, and dismisses many myths on weight loss. It really comes down three things: the PC Score, the PC Score, the PC Score!

CHAPTER 11

SUMMARY

SO, THE PC Diet is a way of losing weight by balancing caloric intake with caloric burn. It stresses the key concept of balancing the value of food with the number of calories it will cost you. The PC Diet aims to maximize protein per calorie consumed (the P/C Ratio). It is a discipline based on understanding how the body stores and burns fat. It's about realizing that you can still eat some "bad" foods and maintain or lose weight. It's about learning how exercise can supplement weight control. And finally, it's not about eating salads every night, protein bars and water for every meal, or worrying about what you eat for every meal. It's about controlling calories, budgeting calories, and making room for calories. It's about asking if that food choice or that extra helping is worth the calories? It's about seeking out foods with the highest amount of protein with the least number of calories (PC Score). And it's about deciding which phase you are in: are you in a weight loss mode, then you need to burn more than you consume in a day; are you in a weight neutral state, matching intake to consumption of calories; but if you are in positive calorie counts more than negative calorie counts, you'll gain weight. It all comes down to the PC Score and balancing your caloric checkbook. You are the best person to design your diet plan, so go get started with your PC Diet and start doing your ACTIVITY OF THE DAY. You've got this!

APPENDIX A:

QUICK ONE PAGE SUMMARY OF THE PC DIET.

1. Consult and follow the advice of your physician before starting any diet. This is only a summary of how I designed a diet for me.
2. Choose an obtainable goal (5-10% of your body weight or 10 lbs for most, as a starter!); Don't over-do it.
3. Choose a time (say 1 month) as your initial trial.
4. Commit and get a support buddy for your mission or challenge a friend, co-worker, or family member.
5. Buy a scale, weigh yourself every morning after emptying your bladder.
6. Maximize your protein in foods you eat during the day, but minimize the calories (Don't waist calories without getting protein)
7. Start calculating the PC Score= Protein/Calories x 100 (PC Score above 5 are great, above 10 is super!)
8. Have a normal dinner (but don't over-eat) each night with your family, friends, or loved ones.
9. Limit your total calories for the day to 1500 for most adults (or 500-1000 under your normal intake for 1-2 lb per week loss, respectively); if want to consume more calories, go burn an extra 500!

10. Remember, water has NO CALORIES; often substituting water for sugar drinks can result in 1 lb loss a week!
11. Calorie check everything you can, stay on budget!
12. Save for over-expenditures and pay-off any over-indulges.
13. Do an Activity of the Day (AOD), every day, even if you only 10-20 minutes; start walking, then jogging, then running! (if cleared by your doctor)
14. Too much protein can be harmful and some people may lack the ability to digest protein, so consult with your doctor prior to this or any diet.
15. Add some fitness to downtime (do pushups on commercials, dumbbell at the office for sets while on the phone, take the stairs, anything to add some fit to your day!
16. Stay hydrated, have fun, and get over that first hill and you've got this!

Protein/calories x 100 = PC Score

Protein (in grams) divided by calories, multiplied by 100

- Enter the grams of protein on any label or menu.
- Divide by the number of calories on any label or menu.
- Multiple by 100.

And REMEMBER,

PC Score Goal: Above 5!

<5:	Bad
5-10:	Good
10-15:	Great
>15:	Super

CPSIA information can be obtained
at www.ICGtesting.com
Printed in the USA
LVHW021502200123
737509LV00002B/584